How to Build Muscle Fast With No Equipment

The At-Home Bible For Cutting Gym Costs and Sculpting a Lean Physique Through Calisthenics and Smart Diet Changes

The Fix-It Guy

Copyright © The Fix-It Guy

Table of Contents

Introduction

Welcome to the thrilling world of muscle building, where sweat, determination, and the burning desire for that sculpted physique collide! If you've ever dreamt of turning your living room into a powerhouse of gains, then congratulations, my friend, you've just stumbled upon the game-changer you've been waiting for.

Picture this: no more awkward gym selfies, no more monthly gym fees that make your wallet cry, and no more waiting for that one guy to finish hogging the bench press. This is the ultimate guide, the At-Home Bible, crafted exclusively for the warriors of change who dare to build muscle without a single piece of traditional equipment. Say goodbye to the clanking of weights, and say hello to a lean, mean home workout routine that will leave you wondering why you ever stepped foot into a gym.

In these pages, we're not just talking about your run-of-the-mill fitness plan; we're diving headfirst into the liberating world of calisthenics, where your body becomes the gym, and every move is a step towards a more powerful, chiseled you. This is not just a book; it's your backstage pass to a fitness revolution, a journey that doesn't just sculpt your muscles but transforms your entire approach to health and well-being.

But hey, don't just take my word for it. Imagine unlocking a world where you can sculpt the physique of your dreams while jamming to your favorite tunes, clad in whatever outrageous workout gear makes you feel unstoppable. It's about embracing the sweat, relishing the burn, and knowing that every drop is an investment in the most important project of your life, YOU.

So, fellow fitness adventurer, if you're ready to bid farewell to the treadmill monotony, if you're eager to redefine your idea of a home workout, and if you're prepared to embrace the at-home muscle-building journey of a lifetime, then buckle up. This isn't just a book; it's your ticket to a stronger, leaner, and more badass version of yourself. Let the gains begin!

Chapter 1

Understanding Calisthenics

What is Calisthenics?

Hey there, fitness explorer! Welcome to the exciting world of calisthenics, where your body becomes the ultimate playground for gains. In this chapter, we'll take a stroll through the basics of calisthenics, ditching the complicated jargon for a conversation that feels like swapping workout tips over a cup of coffee.

What is Calisthenics?

Let's kick things off with a high-five for curiosity! Calisthenics is not some ancient mystical ritual; it's just a fancy word for bodyweight training. Think push-ups, pull-ups, squats, your body, the gym. No fancy equipment, no confusing machines, just you, your muscles, and gravity having a dance party.

The Principles of Bodyweight Training:

1. Your Body, Your Rules: Forget about deciphering cryptic gym machines. With calisthenics, your body weight is the boss. We're talking about natural movements that your body was born to do. Push, pull, squat, it's like going back to the basics, but cooler.

2. Anywhere, Anytime: Imagine this, sculpting those biceps in your living room, abs in the kitchen, and mastering pull-ups at the local park. Calisthenics is the freedom to work out wherever your heart desires. Gym membership? Nah, not necessary.

3. Functional Fitness: Ever wanted to lift groceries with finesse or effortlessly climb stairs like an action hero? Calisthenics not only carves out muscles but makes you a functional fitness ninja in your everyday life.

Why Choose Calisthenics for Muscle Building?

Now, let's talk gains. Why should you swap the bench press for burpees? Here's the lowdown:

1. Whole Body Awesomeness: Calisthenics doesn't discriminate, it works your entire body. No muscle gets left behind. Say hello to a symphony of strength that leaves no stone (or muscle group) unturned.

2. Flexibility to Fit Your Life: Start by choosing the exercises that resonate with you. Hate running but love jumping jacks? Calisthenics is your fitness genie – you decide the moves, the intensity, and the rhythm.

3. Save Your Coins: Gym memberships can be a financial workout in themselves. Calisthenics is the frugal friend of fitness. No need for fancy equipment or pricey memberships, just you and Gravity doing the tango.

Your Action Steps:
1. Pick Three Moves: Choose three calisthenics exercises that make you excited. Push-ups, squats, and lunges are great starters.
2. Set a Date with Your Workout Space: Where's your gym today? Living room, backyard, or local park?

3. Embrace the Soreness: You'll ache a bit. That's your body saying, "Hello, progress!" Embrace it like a badge of honor.

Troubleshooting Tip:
Problem: "I can't do a pull-up!"
Solution: Start with assisted pull-ups using a sturdy chair or resistance bands. Progress at your pace.

So there you have it, the ABCs of calisthenics. Get ready to embrace a workout that not only builds muscles but sets your spirit free. Stay tuned for Chapter 2, where we'll dive into setting goals that make you want to high-five yourself in the mirror. Get ready to crush it!

Chapter 2

Setting Your Goals

Defining Your Fitness Objectives

Hey fitness dreamer! Now that you've dipped your toes into the invigorating world of calisthenics, it's time to set sail on the seas of purpose. Chapter 2 is all about goals, not the kind that involves scoring in a game, but the ones that will leave you feeling like the superhero of your own fitness story.

Defining Your Fitness Objectives

Step 1: Get Clear on Your Why
Start by grabbing a pen and paper (or your trusty digital device) and jot down why you're diving into this calisthenics adventure. Is it to sculpt killer abs, conquer that pull-up, or simply feel more energetic? Your "why" is the North Star guiding you through sweat and soreness.

Troubleshooting Tip:

Problem: "I don't know why I'm doing this."

Solution: Dig deeper. Ask yourself what you want to achieve beyond the physical. Better health? More confidence? Finding your 'why' adds purpose to every push-up.

Step 2: Set SMART Goals

Let's make those dreams tangible. Enter SMART goals, Specific, Measurable, Achievable, Relevant, and Time-Bound. Instead of saying, "I want to get fit," say, "I aim to do 20 push-ups without a break in 4 weeks."

Troubleshooting Tip:

Problem: "My goal feels overwhelming."

Solution: Break it down. If 20 push-ups seem daunting, start with 5 and gradually build up. Small victories lead to big wins.

Step 3: Embrace Variety in Goals

Mix it up! Set short-term and long-term goals. Short-term goals keep you motivated, while long-term goals provide a roadmap. Want to nail that handstand in a month? Fantastic! Dreaming of running a marathon in a year? Let's do it!

Troubleshooting Tip:

Problem: "I'm getting bored with my routine."

Solution: Spice it up. Add new exercises, change your workout location, or challenge a workout buddy. Variety keeps things interesting.

Step 4: Celebrate Non-Scale Victories

Don't be solely scale-focused. Celebrate the victories that can't be measured in pounds. Did you conquer a fear of heights by doing pull-ups? That's a victory. Did you feel more energized throughout the day? Victory, again!

Troubleshooting Tip:

Problem: "I didn't reach my weight goal."

Solution: Reflect on non-scale victories. Improved mood, better sleep, and increased energy are all signs of progress.

Your Action Steps:

1. Draft Your 'Why': Why are you here? What's the burning desire behind your fitness journey?

2. SMART Goals: Write down specific, measurable, achievable, relevant, and time-bound goals.

3. Short-term and Long-term: Mix it up. Set goals you can conquer this month and ones that will keep you inspired over the year.

Congratulations! You've just laid the foundation for a goal-smashing adventure.

Creating Realistic and Achievable Goals

Hey, goal-setter extraordinaire! Now that you're armed with the powerful knowledge of why goals matter, let's roll up our sleeves and make sure those goals are as achievable as a high-five with a friend. In this chapter, we're not just talking about goals; we're talking about goals you can conquer with a fist pump and a grin.

Realistic Goals: Not a Fairy Tale, But Your Story

Step 1: Know Your Starting Point
Before you shoot for the stars, know where you're launching from. Take a fitness selfie (don't worry, it's just for you), jot down how many push-ups you can manage, and be real about your current fitness level. Realistic goals are born from reality, not fantasy.

Troubleshooting Tip:
Problem: "I want to be Superman in a week."
Solution: Superman had his planet. You're doing great on Earth. Set goals that challenge, not crush.

Step 2: Break It Down
Big goals are like a pizza, overwhelming if you try to devour them all at once. Slice them up into bite-sized, achievable pieces. If the ultimate goal is a pizza, then your weekly goals are the slices.

Troubleshooting Tip:

Problem: "I can't eat the whole pizza in one sitting!"

Solution: No one can. Savor each slice. Each workout, each meal, is a step towards the full pie.

Step 3: Flexibility is Key

Life happens. Sometimes you're the windshield, sometimes the bug. Be flexible with your goals. If you miss a workout or indulge in an extra slice of actual pizza, it's okay. Adjust and keep moving forward.

Troubleshooting Tip:

Problem: "I messed up. Might as well quit."

Solution: Nope. You stumbled, not fell. Get up, dust off, and keep going.

Tracking Progress Without Traditional Gym Equipment

Now, let's address the elephant in the room, the lack of shiny gym equipment. Who needs it anyway? We're calisthenics warriors, and our progress is measured in push-ups, not dumbbells.

Step 1: The Power of Repetition

Count your reps, not the minutes on a treadmill. Whether it's push-ups, squats, or burpees, track the number you can do in a set. Progress may start to slow, but it's the steady climb that gets you to the summit.

Troubleshooting Tip:

Problem: "I'm not seeing progress."

Solution: Keep a workout journal. Seeing the numbers on paper is like watching your own superhero origin story.

Step 2: Time and Intensity Matter

Clock your workouts. How long does it take you to complete a routine? Are you pushing yourself a bit more each time? Time and intensity are your secret weapons, and they don't require a fancy gym clock.

Troubleshooting Tip:

Problem: "I'm not feeling challenged."

Solution: Shorten rest periods or add a more challenging variation. The burn is your progress handshake.

Your Action Steps:

1. **Real Talk with Yourself:** Where are you starting from? Be honest.

2. **Slice It Up:** Break your big goals into bite-sized, achievable pieces.

3. **Be Flexible:** Life is a rollercoaster. Enjoy the ride, bumps, and all.

You're on the path to goal-setting glory! Chapter 3 is just around the corner, where we'll explore the world of nutrition, because a well-fed warrior is a powerful one. Get ready to unleash your inner food ninja!

Chapter 3

The Basics of Nutrition

Fueling Your Body for Muscle Growth

Hey, nutrition navigator! Welcome to the kitchen, where the real gains are cooked up. Chapter 3 is your backstage pass to understanding the fuel that will turn your calisthenics journey into a muscle-building symphony. So, grab a fork, and let's dive into the delicious world of nutrition!

Fueling Your Body for Muscle Growth

Step 1: Embrace the Protein Party
Protein is your muscle's best friend. It's like the bouncer at the club, it repairs and builds. Chicken, eggs, beans, and Greek yogurt are the VIPs on this guest list. Aim for protein in every meal, and your muscles will thank you.

Troubleshooting Tip:
Problem: "I'm tired of chicken."
Solution: Mix it up! Try fish, tofu, or plant-based proteins. Your taste buds will thank you.

Step 2: Carbs: Not the Enemy, But the Ally

Carbs are the energy ninjas that fuel your workouts. Opt for complex carbs like sweet potatoes, whole grains, and oats. They're the slow-burning fuel that keeps you going through those burpees and squats.

Troubleshooting Tip:

Problem: "Carbs make me bloated."

Solution: Drink more water and choose fiber-rich carbs. Your digestive system will be doing cartwheels.

Step 3: Don't Forget the Good Fats

Fat is not the villain; it's the hero your body needs. Avocados, nuts, and olive oil are like the Avengers of fats. They support hormone production and keep your joints lubricated.

Troubleshooting Tip:

Problem: "I'm scared of fats."

Solution: Don't be! Embrace the good fats in moderation. They're the sidekick your body deserves.*

Step 4: Hydration, the Unsung Hero

Water is the silent MVP of your fitness journey. It keeps you hydrated, aids digestion, and supports overall well-being. Aim for at least eight glasses a day, and your body will thank you with optimal performance.

Troubleshooting Tip:

Problem: "I forget to drink water."

Solution: Set reminders on your phone, carry a water bottle, or infuse your water with fruits for a tasty twist.

Your Action Steps:

1. Protein Palooza: Include a good protein source in every meal.

2. Carb Conscious: Opt for complex carbs to fuel your workouts.

3. Fat Friends: Embrace the good fats, they're on your team.

4. Hydration Station: Drink water like it's your job.

Congratulations! You've just earned your nutrition black belt.

Building a Muscle-Friendly Diet

Hey, culinary architect! Now that we've established the importance of the right fuel, let's get down to crafting a diet that turns your kitchen into a muscle-building haven. In this chapter, we're not just talking about eating; we're talking about creating a symphony of nutrients that will have your muscles singing a powerful anthem of growth.

The Foundation: Protein Paradise

Step 1: Protein Prowess

Protein isn't just a guest at the party; it's the headliner. Whether it's grilled chicken, eggs, lentils, or that post-workout protein shake, make sure your plate is rocking a generous serving of muscle-building goodness.

Troubleshooting Tip:

Problem: "I'm a vegetarian."

Solution: Hello, plant-based proteins! Quinoa, tofu, and beans are your new best friends.

Building Blocks: Carbs, the Right Way

Step 2: Carb Construction

Carbs are the architects of energy. Opt for complex carbs like brown rice, sweet potatoes, and whole-grain bread.

They're the steady builders that keep your energy levels soaring throughout the day.

Troubleshooting Tip:
Problem: "I thought carbs are bad."
Solution: Nah, it's the processed stuff that's the party crasher. Stick to the whole, unprocessed carbs for a dance party in your body.

The Finishing Touch: Healthy Fats

Step 3: Fat Flourish
Fats are the artists that add flavor to the masterpiece. Avocados, nuts, and olive oil not only make your meals tasty but also support hormone production and overall body function.

Troubleshooting Tip:
Problem: "I'm on a low-fat diet."
Solution: Your body needs fats, the good kind. Keep it balanced and let those good fats play their role.

Hydration Oasis: The Silent Performer

Step 4: Water Wonderland
Water isn't just a drink; it's the backstage manager ensuring everything runs smoothly. Hydration is key for

digestion, nutrient absorption, and overall performance. Make it a habit to keep that water bottle by your side.

Troubleshooting Tip:
Problem: "Water is boring."
Solution: Infuse it! Drop in some berries, cucumber, or mint for a refreshing twist.

Your Action Steps:
1. **Protein Power-Up:** Incorporate lean protein sources into every meal.
2. **Carb Crafting:** Choose complex carbs for sustained energy.
3. **Fats in Harmony:** Include healthy fats for flavor and overall health.
4. **Hydration Habits:** Drink water like it's your elixir.

Congratulations! You've just designed a menu that's not just tasty but a powerhouse for muscle growth.

Nutrient Timing and Its Impact on Results

Hey, time traveler of nutrients! In this chapter, we're diving into the fascinating world of when to eat what, because timing isn't just crucial in comedy, it's a game-changer in the realm of muscle-building. So, grab your fork, and let's synchronize your meals for maximum impact!

The Prelude: Breakfast, the Kickstart

Step 1: Breakfast Brilliance
Breakfast isn't just a meal; it's your morning battle cry. Kickstart your day with a balance of protein, carbs, and fats. Whether it's eggs, oatmeal, or a smoothie, make sure it's a powerhouse to fuel your morning exploits.

Troubleshooting Tip:
Problem: "I'm not a morning eater."
Solution: Start small, a piece of fruit, yogurt, or a handful of nuts. Your body will thank you for the morning nudge.

The Intermission: Pre-Workout Nutrition

Step 2: Pre-Workout Power-Up

Your body needs fuel before the workout symphony begins. Aim for a light meal or snack about 1-2 hours before exercising. Think bananas, yogurt, or a small sandwich. It's the energy boost you need without feeling weighed down.

Troubleshooting Tip:

Problem: "I work out on an empty stomach."
Solution: A small snack won't sabotage your workout. It'll enhance it. Try a banana or a handful of almonds.

The Climax: Post-Workout Refuel

Step 3: Post-Workout Replenishment

After the workout finale, your body craves replenishment. Aim to refuel within 30-60 minutes with a mix of protein and carbs. This could be a protein shake, Greek yogurt with berries, or a turkey sandwich. It's the recovery anthem your muscles need.

Troubleshooting Tip:

Problem: "I don't feel hungry after a workout."
Solution: You don't have to be starving. Even a small snack can kickstart the recovery process.

The Resolution: Evening Eats

Step 4: Dinner Delight

Dinner isn't just a conclusion; it's the resolution to a day of hard work. Opt for a balanced meal with lean protein, veggies, and complex carbs. Grilled chicken, quinoa, and a colorful array of veggies, now that's a dinner worth celebrating.

Troubleshooting Tip:

Problem: "I crave late-night snacks."

Solution: Snack wisely. Greek yogurt, a small handful of nuts, or a piece of fruit can satisfy without derailing your efforts.

Your Action Steps:

1. **Breakfast Boost:** Fuel your morning with a balanced breakfast.

2. **Pre-Workout Prep:** Snack wisely before your workout for sustained energy.

3. **Post-Workout Recharge:** Refuel within an hour of your workout with a mix of protein and carbs.

4. **Dinner Decisions:** Conclude your day with a balanced, nutrient-rich dinner.

Congratulations! You've just mastered the art of nutrient timing, turning your meals into strategic maneuvers for optimal results.

Chapter 4

No-Equipment Workouts

Designing Effective Home Workouts

Hey, home workout hero! In this chapter, we're breaking free from the shackles of gym equipment and transforming your living space into a powerhouse of gains. No dumbbells, no fancy machines, just you, your determination, and the thrill of sculpting your body without leaving the comfort of home. Let's dive into the exciting world of no-equipment workouts!

Unleashing Your Inner Warrior

Step 1: Master the Basics
Before we craft your no-equipment symphony, let's brush up on the basics. Mastering fundamental movements like squats, lunges, push-ups, and planks lays the foundation for a workout that hits all the right notes. No PhD in Exercise Science is required, just your body and a willingness to move.

Troubleshooting Tip:
Problem: "I can't do a proper push-up."

Solution: Start with incline push-ups or wall push-ups. Gradually, as you get stronger, move to the floor.

Designing Your Workout Routine

Step 2: Mix and Match Movements

Your home workout, your rules. Mix and match movements to target different muscle groups. Start with a warm-up of jumping jacks or high knees, then dive into a circuit of bodyweight exercises. Squats, lunges, and push-ups can form the backbone, with mountain climbers and burpees for that extra spice.

Troubleshooting Tip:

Problem: "I get bored easily."

Solution: Get creative! Add music, change up the order of exercises, or explore new variations. The more fun, the better.

Introducing the Element of Progress

Step 3: Progressive Overload at Home

Who needs weights when you have the power of progress? Increase the intensity gradually. Add more reps, reduce rest time, or try advanced variations of exercises. Your muscles crave a challenge, and progressive overload is the secret sauce.

Troubleshooting Tip:
Problem: "It's too easy now."
Solution: Amp it up! Increase the intensity, try more challenging variations, or add explosive movements for that extra burn.

Tailoring Your Routine to You

Step 4: Personalize Your Plan
Your body, your rules, your goals. Tailor your routine to fit your fitness level and aspirations. If you're a beginner, start with simpler exercises and gradually level up. If you're a seasoned warrior, push your limits and embrace the burn.

Troubleshooting Tip:
Problem: "I don't have much time."
Solution: Quality over quantity. A short, intense workout can be as effective as a longer one. Squeeze it into your schedule.

Your Action Steps:
1. Master the Basics: Nail fundamental movements like squats, lunges, and push-ups.
2. Mix and Match: Design a circuit of bodyweight exercises targeting different muscle groups.
3. Progressive Overload: Challenge yourself by increasing intensity over time.

4. Personalize Your Plan: Tailor your routine to your fitness level and goals.

Congratulations! You're now the architect of your home workout destiny. In Chapter 5, we'll address the advanced techniques and ninja moves of calisthenics. Get ready to unlock the next level of bodyweight mastery!

Targeting Different Muscle Groups

Hello muscle maestro! Now that you've embraced the no-equipment ethos, it's time to become a sculptor, chiseling away at different muscle groups. In this chapter, we're going to play the symphony of calisthenics, hitting every muscle from head to toe. Get ready to unleash the beast within as we delve into the art of targeting different muscle groups without a single piece of traditional gym equipment!

The Core Conductor: Abs and Lower Back

Step 1: Abs of Steel

Let's start with the epicenter of strength, your core. Planks, mountain climbers, and leg raises are your go-to moves. These exercises not only carve out a six-pack but also fortify your lower back. Your core is not just for show; it's the powerhouse that fuels every move.

Troubleshooting Tip:

Problem: "Crunches hurt my neck."

Solution: Opt for alternative core exercises like planks or Russian twists. Your core will still get the love.

The Upper Symphony: Chest, Shoulders, and Arms

Step 2: Sculpted Upper Body

Time to focus on that impressive upper deck. Push-ups, dips, and pike push-ups will be your main players. They engage your chest, shoulders, triceps, and even a bit of that sneaky core. It's the recipe for a strong, well-defined upper body without a single dumbbell in sight.

Troubleshooting Tip:

Problem: "Push-ups are too easy."

Solution: Elevate your feet or try one-arm push-ups. The burn will come knocking.

The Mighty Pillars: Legs and Glutes

Step 3: Leg Day Nirvana

Leg Day doesn't need a squat rack. Master the art of bodyweight squats, lunges, and step-ups. These exercises target your quads, hamstrings, and glutes, turning your legs into pillars of strength. Your staircase is now your stairway to gains.

Troubleshooting Tip:

Problem: "I don't feel the burn in my glutes."

Solution: Go deeper in your squats, focus on the squeeze at the top, and add glute bridges for that extra burn.

The Stealth Warriors: Back and Lats

Step 4: Backyard Back Workout

No equipment, no problem. Activate those back muscles with exercises like inverted rows, Superman lifts, and doorway pull-ups. Your back and lats are the unsung heroes, supporting your posture and giving you that confident, superhero stance.

Troubleshooting Tip:

Problem: "Pull-ups are impossible."

Solution: Start with inverted rows and gradually progress. You'll be hanging like a monkey in no time.

Your Action Steps:

1. Core Command: Planks, mountain climbers, and leg raises for a rock-solid core.

2. Upper Elevation: Push-ups, dips, and pike push-ups for a sculpted upper body.

3. Leg Luminary: Bodyweight squats, lunges, and step-ups for powerful legs.

4. Backyard Bliss: Inverted rows, Superman lifts, and doorway pull-ups for a strong back.

Congratulations! You've just orchestrated a full-body workout without a single piece of equipment. In the next Chapter, we'll explore advanced calisthenics techniques to take your bodyweight mastery to the next level. Get ready for the ninja moves of the calisthenics world!

Incorporating Progressive Overload

Greetings, fitness alchemist! Now that you've mastered the basics, let's sprinkle a bit of magic into your routine. In this chapter, we're delving into the transformative art of progressive overload, a key ingredient that turns a good workout into a muscle-sculpting masterpiece. Get ready to ascend to new heights as we explore the world of challenging your body and unlocking its true potential without fancy equipment.

The Magic of Progression

Step 1: Reps, Sets, and Beyond
Progressive overload is the secret sauce that keeps your muscles guessing and growing. Begin by manipulating reps and sets. Increase the number of repetitions or add an extra set to your exercises as your strength improves. This gradual escalation keeps your muscles on their toes, adapting and growing in response to the increasing demands.

Troubleshooting Tip:
Problem: "I'm stuck at the same reps."
Solution: Break through the plateau by increasing reps incrementally. Your muscles thrive on gentle challenges.

The Weightless Challenge

Step 2: Adding Difficulty Sans Weights

Who needs dumbbells when you can make bodyweight exercises more challenging? Elevate your feet during push-ups, opt for one-legged squats, or explore explosive movements like jump squats and explosive push-ups. The absence of weights doesn't mean the absence of resistance, make your muscles work harder against gravity.

Troubleshooting Tip:
Problem: "Standard squats are getting too easy."
Solution: Upgrade to one-legged squats or try pistol squats. Your balance and strength will thank you.

The Time Under Tension Technique

Step 3: Slow and Steady Wins the Race

Introduce the concept of time under tension to your routine. Slow down the pace of your exercises, whether it's a slow descent during a squat or a deliberate push during a push-up. This not only intensifies the workout but also engages your muscles for longer, promoting growth and strength.

Troubleshooting Tip:
Problem: "I rush through my exercises."

Solution: Embrace the art of controlled movements. Slowing down ensures every rep counts.

The Variable Rest Period

Step 4: Mix Up the Rest Intervals

The time you rest between sets is a variable that can influence the difficulty of your workout. Shorten the rest periods to keep your heart rate up and intensify the workout. Alternatively, lengthen the rest periods when aiming for maximum strength. The key is to adapt the rest intervals to your specific fitness goals.

Troubleshooting Tip:

Problem: "I rest too long between sets."
Solution: Set a timer. Whether it's 30 seconds or 90 seconds, stick to it. The clock is your workout buddy.

Your Action Steps:

1. Reps and Sets Roulette: Gradually increase the number of reps or sets to challenge your muscles.
2. Weightless Resistance: Elevate exercises or introduce explosive movements for added difficulty.
3. Time Under Tension: Slow down the pace of your exercises to engage muscles for longer.
4. Rest Period Variability: Adjust rest intervals based on your fitness goals.

Congratulations! You've just unlocked the door to continual progress and growth. In Chapter 4, we'll delve into advanced calisthenics techniques that will have you performing feats you once thought impossible. Get ready to unleash your inner ninja!

Chapter 5

Advanced Calisthenics Techniques

Mastering Bodyweight Exercises

Greetings, aspiring calisthenics virtuoso! In this chapter, we're diving into the realm of advanced techniques that will elevate your bodyweight workouts to new heights. Brace yourself for a journey that goes beyond the basics, unlocking the secrets of mastering advanced bodyweight exercises. Get ready to soar like a calisthenics ninja!

The Handstand Symphony

1. Handstand Push-Ups:

Execution:
1. Start in a handstand position against a wall.
2. Lower your body toward the ground by bending your elbows.
3. Push back up to the starting position.
4. Maintain a straight body throughout the movement.

Tips:

- Engage your core to keep your body aligned.
- Gradually increase the depth of your push-ups as strength builds.

The Human Flag Extravaganza

2. Human Flag:

Execution:

1. Grasp a vertical object (like a pole) with both hands.
2. Lift your body horizontally, keeping it parallel to the ground.
3. Legs should be straight and body tight.
4. Engage your core and hold the position.

Tips:

- Start with tuck flags and progress to straight legs.
- Practice against a sturdy support until your strength improves.

The Gravity-Defying Muscle-Up

3. Muscle-Up Mastery:

Execution:

1. Begin with a hanging position on a bar.

2. Explosively pull yourself up, transitioning to a dip position.
3. Push up to complete the movement.
4. Lower back down with control.

Tips:

- Master pull-ups and dips before attempting muscle-ups.
- Use a false grip for a smoother transition over the bar.

The Elegant L-Sit

4. L-Sit Perfection:

Execution:
1. Sit on the ground with your legs extended.
2. Place your hands beside your hips and lift your body.
3. Keep legs straight, forming an 'L' shape.
4. Hold for the desired duration.

Tips:

- Start with one-foot support and progress to full L-sits.
- Engage your core to lift your legs higher.

The Explosive Plyometric Clap Push-Up

5. Clap Push-Up Explosion:

Execution:
1. Begin with a standard push-up position.
2. Lower your body to the ground.
3. Explosively push up, clapping your hands together.
4. Land with control and repeat.

Tips:
- Focus on explosive power.
- Land with slightly bent elbows to absorb impact.

Your Action Steps:

1. Handstand Hustle: Practice handstand push-ups against a wall.
2. Flag Flow: Begin with tuck flags before progressing to full human flags.
3. Muscle-Up Mastery: Build strength with pull-ups and dips.
4. L-Sit Launch: Progress from one-foot support to a full L-sit.
5. Clap Push-Up Challenge: Master explosive power with clap push-ups.

Increasing Intensity Without Weights

Hello intensity seeker! In this chapter, we're diving into the art of turning up the heat on your workouts without the need for bulky weights. Whether you're a bodyweight purist or simply working out at home, these techniques will set your muscles on fire and take your fitness journey to a whole new level. Get ready to crank up the intensity and break through plateaus without a single dumbbell in sight!

The Power of Progression

1. Increase Repetitions:

Strategy:
- Gradually add more repetitions to your exercises.
- Push your limits without compromising form.

Troubleshooting Tip:
Problem: "I can't do more reps."
Solution: Aim for one more rep than your previous workout. Slowly, the numbers will climb.

The Tempo Twist

2. Slow Down the Pace:

Strategy:

- Embrace slow, controlled movements for each exercise.
- Increase the time under tension to intensify the workout.

Troubleshooting Tip:

Problem: "I rush through my exercises."

Solution: Count to three on the way down and three on the way up. Quality over quantity!

The Circuit Surge

3. Create High-Intensity Circuits:

Strategy:

- Combine different exercises into a circuit.
- Minimal rest between exercises to keep the heart rate up.

Troubleshooting Tip:

Problem: "Circuits are too tiring."

Solution: Start with a shorter circuit and gradually increase the duration as your stamina improves.

The Super Set Challenge

4. Super Set Your Exercises:

Strategy:

- Pair two exercises targeting different muscle groups.
- Perform them back-to-back with minimal rest.

Troubleshooting Tip:

Problem: "I'm not feeling the burn."

Solution: Choose exercises that complement each other and focus on muscle fatigue.

The Elevated Challenge

5. Elevate Your Movements:

Strategy:

- Increase the difficulty of exercises by elevating your feet or hands.
- This adds resistance and engages more muscle fibers.

Troubleshooting Tip:

Problem: "Elevated exercises are too hard."

Solution: Start with a lower elevation and progressively increase as your strength improves.

Your Action Steps:

1. Rep Revelry: Gradually increase repetitions for each exercise.

2. Tempo Transformation: Slow down the pace for controlled movements.

3. Circuit Symphony: Create high-intensity circuits for a full-body burn.

4. Super Set Showdown: Pair complementary exercises with minimal rest.

5. Elevated Excellence: Increase difficulty by elevating your movements.

Overcoming Plateaus with Creative Techniques

Hello plateau buster! In this chapter, we're diving into the creative and unconventional techniques that will shatter the walls of stagnation. Whether you've hit a roadblock in your progress or just want to keep things fresh, these strategies will inject new life into your workouts. Say goodbye to plateaus and hello to progress!

The Challenge of Unpredictability

1. Randomize Your Routine:

Strategy:
- Shuffle your exercises like a deck of cards.
- Let chance dictate your workout sequence.

Troubleshooting Tip:
Problem: "I like routine."
Solution: Embrace the chaos! The unpredictability keeps your body guessing.

The Environment Switch-Up

2. Take It Outdoors:

Strategy:

- Move your workout to a park, beach, or any outdoor space.
- Utilize natural elements like rocks or benches.

Troubleshooting Tip:
Problem: "I prefer the gym."
Solution: Nature is your new gym. Fresh air and sunlight can be powerful motivators.

The Technique Twist

3. Embrace Unconventional Movements:

Strategy:

- Integrate animal movements (bear crawls, crab walks) into your routine.
- Incorporate dance or martial arts-inspired sequences.

Troubleshooting Tip:
Problem: "It feels silly."
Solution: Unconventional doesn't mean ineffective. Have fun and let your body explore new ranges of motion.

The Hybrid Fusion

4. Blend Different Disciplines:

Strategy:
- Combine elements from yoga, Pilates, and calisthenics.
- Create hybrid workouts that challenge your body in new ways.

Troubleshooting Tip:
Problem: "I'm not flexible enough."
Solution: Flexibility comes with practice. Enjoy the journey of learning new skills.

The Mind-Body Connection

5. Incorporate Mindful Movements:

Strategy:
- Introduce mindfulness practices like tai chi or qigong.
- Connect your movements with your breath and focus.

Troubleshooting Tip:
Problem: "I don't have time for mindfulness."

Solution: A few minutes of mindfulness can enhance your overall well-being and break mental plateaus.

Your Action Steps:

1. Random Routine Roulette: Let chance dictate your workout sequence.

2. Outdoor Odyssey: Take your workout to the great outdoors.

3. Unconventional Universe: Explore animal movements and unconventional exercises.

4. Discipline Fusion: Blend elements from different disciplines for a diverse workout.

5. Mindful Motion: Incorporate mindful practices to enhance mind-body connection.

Chapter 6

Recovery and Rest

Importance of Rest in Muscle Building

Greetings, recovery enthusiast! In this chapter, we'll unravel the essential role of rest in the intricate dance of muscle building. As much as we love the thrill of a challenging workout, it's during the moments of rest that our bodies truly transform. So, kick back, relax, and let's explore the crucial importance of recovery in sculpting the physique of your dreams.

The Rejuvenating Power of Rest

1. Muscle Repair and Growth:

Insight:
- Rest is not just a break; it's the magic potion for muscle recovery.
- During rest, microscopic muscle fibers damaged during workouts repair and grow stronger.

Troubleshooting Tip:
Problem: "I feel guilty about resting."

Solution: Embrace rest as an active part of your fitness journey. It's not slacking off; it's smart training.

The Hormonal Harmony

2. Balancing Hormones:

Insight:

- Adequate rest helps regulate hormones like cortisol and testosterone.
- Cortisol, the stress hormone, decreases during rest, while testosterone, essential for muscle growth, gets a boost.

Troubleshooting Tip:
Problem: "I'm stressed all the time."
Solution: Prioritize sleep, meditation, and relaxation techniques to keep stress hormones in check.

The Energy Bank Refill

3. Replenishing Energy Reserves:

Insight:

- Rest allows your body to replenish glycogen stores.
- Adequate glycogen levels are crucial for sustained energy during workouts.

Troubleshooting Tip:
Problem: "I always feel drained."
Solution: Ensure you're getting enough sleep and consuming a balanced diet to support energy replenishment.

The Mental Recharge

4. Cognitive Restoration:

Insight:
- Rest is not just for the body; it's a boon for the mind.
- Quality sleep enhances cognitive function, focus, and decision-making.

Troubleshooting Tip:
Problem: "I'm always mentally fatigued."
Solution: Prioritize sleep hygiene and incorporate activities like meditation to recharge your mental batteries.

The Injury Prevention Shield

5. Preventing Burnout and Injuries:

Insight:

- Overtraining increases the risk of burnout and injuries.
- Adequate rest provides the necessary recovery time, reducing the likelihood of both.

Troubleshooting Tip:

Problem: "I want faster results."

Solution: Patience is a virtue. Consistent, balanced training with ample rest yields sustainable results.

Your Action Steps:

1. Strategic Sleep: Prioritize quality sleep for optimal recovery.

2. Active Rest Days: Incorporate light activities on rest days, like walking or yoga.

3. Nutrient-Rich Diet: Fuel your body with a balanced diet to support recovery.

4. Hydration Habits: Maintain proper hydration levels for overall well-being.

5. Mindful Recovery: Incorporate mindfulness practices for mental rejuvenation.

Congratulations! You've now unlocked the secrets of the crucial role of recovery and rest in the muscle-building journey.

Incorporating Rest Days into Your Routine

Hey, rest champion! In this chapter, we're diving into the art of intentional rest, the secret sauce that propels your fitness journey forward. Rest days aren't just breaks; they're strategic moves in the grand chessboard of muscle building. Let's explore how to weave these crucial rest days into your routine for optimal results.

The Purposeful Pause

1. Understanding Rest's Role:

Insight:
- Rest days are not a sign of weakness; they're a strategic necessity.
- They allow your muscles to repair, grow, and come back stronger.

Troubleshooting Tip:
Problem: "I feel guilty on rest days."
Solution: Rest is a part of the process, not a detour. Embrace it.

The Rest Frequency Dance

2. Tailoring Rest Frequency:

Strategy:

- Plan regular rest days based on your workout intensity.
- Beginners might benefit from more frequent rest, while advanced athletes can space them out.

Troubleshooting Tip:

Problem: "How many rest days do I need?"

Solution: Listen to your body. If you're feeling fatigued or experiencing persistent soreness, it might be time for a rest day.

The Active Recovery Ballet

3. Incorporating Active Recovery:

Strategy:

- Engage in light activities on rest days.
- Gentle exercises like walking, yoga, or swimming promote blood flow without taxing your muscles.

Troubleshooting Tip:

Problem: "I feel restless on rest days."

Solution: Turn rest days into active recovery days. It's a win-win for your body and mind.

The Sleep Sanctuary

4. Prioritizing Sleep:

Strategy:
- Make sleep a non-negotiable part of your recovery plan.
- Quality sleep is when your body undergoes significant repair and growth.

Troubleshooting Tip:
Problem: "I struggle to sleep well."
Solution: Create a sleep-friendly environment, limit screen time before bed, and establish a consistent sleep schedule.

The Nutrition Recharge

5. Optimizing Nutrition on Rest Days:

Strategy:
- Adjust your nutrition on rest days to support recovery.
- Focus on adequate protein, hydration, and nutrient-rich foods.

Troubleshooting Tip:
Problem: "I lose my appetite on rest days."

Solution: Opt for smaller, nutrient-dense meals and stay hydrated to support recovery.

Your Action Steps:

1. Rest Day Blueprint: Plan strategic rest days into your weekly routine.

2. Active Recovery Choices: Incorporate light activities on rest days.

3. Sleep Sanctuary: Prioritize quality sleep for optimal recovery.

4. Nutrient Optimization: Adjust your nutrition to support recovery on rest days.

5. Mindful Rest: Embrace rest days as a vital part of your fitness journey.

Overcoming Plateaus with Creative Techniques

Hello plateau buster! In this chapter, we're diving into the creative and unconventional techniques that will shatter the walls of stagnation. Whether you've hit a roadblock in your progress or just want to keep things fresh, these strategies will inject new life into your workouts. Say goodbye to plateaus and hello to progress!

The Challenge of Unpredictability

1. Randomize Your Routine:

Strategy:
- Shuffle your exercises like a deck of cards.
- Let chance dictate your workout sequence.

Troubleshooting Tip:
Problem: "I like routine."
Solution: Embrace the chaos! The unpredictability keeps your body guessing.

The Environment Switch-Up

2. Take It Outdoors:

Strategy:
- Move your workout to a park, beach, or any outdoor space.
- Utilize natural elements like rocks or benches.

Troubleshooting Tip:
Problem: "I prefer the gym."
Solution: Nature is your new gym. Fresh air and sunlight can be powerful motivators.

The Technique Twist

3. Embrace Unconventional Movements:

Strategy:
- Integrate animal movements (bear crawls, crab walks) into your routine.
- Incorporate dance or martial arts-inspired sequences.

Troubleshooting Tip:
Problem: "It feels silly."

Solution: Unconventional doesn't mean ineffective. Have fun and let your body explore new ranges of motion.

The Hybrid Fusion

4. Blend Different Disciplines:

Strategy:

- Combine elements from yoga, Pilates, and calisthenics.
- Create hybrid workouts that challenge your body in new ways.

Troubleshooting Tip:
Problem: "I'm not flexible enough."
Solution: Flexibility comes with practice. Enjoy the journey of learning new skills.

The Mind-Body Connection

5. Incorporate Mindful Movements:

Strategy:

- Introduce mindfulness practices like tai chi or qigong.
- Connect your movements with your breath and focus.

Troubleshooting Tip:

Problem: "I don't have time for mindfulness."

Solution: A few minutes of mindfulness can enhance your overall well-being and break mental plateaus.

Your Action Steps:

1. Random Routine Roulette: Let chance dictate your workout sequence.

2. Outdoor Odyssey: Take your workout to the great outdoors.

3. Unconventional Universe: Explore animal movements and unconventional exercises.

4. Discipline Fusion: Blend elements from different disciplines for a diverse workout.

5. Mindful Motion: Incorporate mindful practices to enhance mind-body connection.

Sleep and its Role in Muscle Recovery

Hello sleep seeker! In this chapter, we're delving into the often underestimated, yet paramount, pillar of your fitness journey, sleep. It's not just a nightly routine; it's the backstage pass to muscle recovery and overall well-being. So, let's uncover the profound influence of quality sleep on your body's ability to rebuild, rejuvenate, and sculpt the physique of your dreams.

The Regenerative Power of Sleep

1. Nightly Repair and Growth:

Insight:
- Sleep is your body's prime time for repair and growth.
- During the deeper stages of sleep, the pituitary gland releases growth hormone, essential for muscle recovery.

Troubleshooting Tip:
Problem: "I struggle to get enough sleep."
Solution: Prioritize sleep like a crucial appointment. Create a relaxing pre-sleep routine to signal to your body that it's time to wind down.

The Hormonal Harmony Symphony

2. Cortisol Control and Testosterone Boost:

Insight:

- A good night's sleep helps regulate cortisol, the stress hormone.
- Optimal sleep supports the release of testosterone, a key player in muscle development.

Troubleshooting Tip:
Problem: "I'm stressed, even in bed."
Solution: Incorporate relaxation techniques before bedtime, such as deep breathing or gentle stretching.

The Memory Lane of Muscle Movements

3. Memory Consolidation for Motor Skills:

Insight:

- During sleep, your brain consolidates memories, including motor skills learned during your workouts.
- Quality sleep enhances the retention of exercise techniques and movements.

Troubleshooting Tip:

Problem: "I forget workout techniques easily."

Solution: Review and visualize your workout routine before bedtime to enhance memory consolidation.

The Immune System Guardian

4. Immune System Fortification:

Insight:

- Adequate sleep strengthens your immune system.
- A robust immune system is crucial for overall health and sustained workout consistency.

Troubleshooting Tip:

Problem: "I catch every bug going around."

Solution: Prioritize sleep hygiene to give your immune system the support it needs.

The Pain Perception Dimmer

5. Pain Perception Management:

Insight:

- Sleep influences your pain perception.
- Quality sleep can reduce the perception of pain and discomfort, aiding recovery from intense workouts.

Troubleshooting Tip:
Problem: "I wake up sore every day."
Solution: Ensure your sleep environment is comfortable and invest in a supportive mattress and pillows.

Your Action Steps:

1. Sleep Sanctuary Setup: Create a sleep-friendly environment for optimal rest.

2. Consistent Sleep Schedule: Establish a consistent bedtime routine to regulate your body's internal clock.

3. Digital Detox Before Bed: Limit screen time before sleep to promote relaxation.

4. Mindfulness Practices: Incorporate relaxation techniques like meditation or gentle stretching.

5. Sleep Quantity and Quality: Aim for 7-9 hours of quality sleep each night for optimal recovery.

Congratulations! You've now unlocked the secrets of how sleep plays a pivotal role in muscle recovery and overall well-being. In the final chapter, we'll explore effective goal-setting strategies and discuss the keys to maintaining a lifelong commitment to your well-being. Get ready to seal the deal on your fitness success!

Chapter 7

Troubleshooting Common Challenges

Dealing with Plateaus

Hey troubleshooter! In this chapter, we're tackling one of the most common adversaries in the fitness world, plateaus. These frustrating plateaus can feel like hitting a brick wall, but fear not! We'll explore effective strategies to smash through these barriers and reignite the flames of progress. Let's dive into the art of troubleshooting plateaus and reclaiming the momentum in your muscle-building journey.

The Plateau Plague

1. Understanding Plateaus:

Insight:
- Plateaus are a natural part of any fitness journey.
- They often occur when the body adapts to a specific workout routine, leading to a slowdown in progress.

Troubleshooting Tip:

Problem: "I'm stuck in a rut."

Solution: Shift your perspective. Plateaus are not roadblocks; they're signals to reassess and adjust your approach.

The Variety Vortex

2. Introducing Workout Variety:

Strategy:

- Shake up your routine by introducing new exercises and variations.
- Novel stimuli challenge your muscles in different ways, breaking through plateaus.

Troubleshooting Tip:

Problem: "I'm bored with my routine."

Solution: Embrace variety. Try new exercises, change your workout order, or explore different training styles.

The Progressive Overload Puzzle

3. Revisiting Progressive Overload:

Strategy:

- Reassess your progressive overload strategy.

- Increase intensity, adjust rep ranges, or try advanced variations to challenge your muscles.

Troubleshooting Tip:

Problem: "My workouts feel too easy."

Solution: Up the ante. Your muscles thrive on the principle of progressive overload, give them a reason to grow.

The Recovery Renaissance

4. Prioritizing Recovery:

Strategy:
- Ensure you're getting adequate rest between workouts.
- Explore active recovery techniques and consider deloading periods.

Troubleshooting Tip:

Problem: "I'm always fatigued."

Solution: Evaluate your sleep quality, nutrition, and stress levels. Recovery is as crucial as the workouts themselves.

The Nutrition Nudge

5. *Optimizing Nutrition for Breakthroughs:*

Strategy:
- Reevaluate your nutritional intake to support your goals.
- Ensure you're getting enough protein, carbs, and healthy fats.

Troubleshooting Tip:
Problem: "My diet is off-track."
Solution: Dial in your nutrition. Consult with a nutritionist if needed to align your diet with your fitness goals.

Your Action Steps:

1. Routine Remix: Introduce new exercises and variations into your routine.
2. Intensity Injection: Reassess and increase the intensity of your workouts.
3. Recovery Revamp: Prioritize quality sleep, active recovery, and deload periods.
4. Nutrition Tune-Up: Evaluate and optimize your nutritional intake.
5. Mindset Reset: Embrace plateaus as opportunities for growth and change.

Adapting Workouts to Personal Limitations

Hello injury navigator! In this chapter, we're diving into the delicate but crucial territory of handling common injuries and strains. Whether you've encountered a minor setback or are dealing with a persistent discomfort, we'll explore effective strategies to address, adapt, and overcome. Let's embark on a journey of resilience, adapting workouts to your limitations, and ensuring a safe path forward in your muscle-building adventure.

The Injury Insight

1. Understanding Common Injuries:

Insight:
- Injuries and strains are not uncommon in the fitness journey.
- Common culprits include muscle strains, tendonitis, and joint discomfort.

Troubleshooting Tip:
Problem: "I'm dealing with pain."
Solution: Listen to your body. Persistent pain is a signal to pause, assess, and take action.

The Art of Modification

2. Adapting Workouts to Limitations:

Strategy:
- Modify exercises to accommodate your limitations.
- Focus on movements that don't aggravate the injured area.

Troubleshooting Tip:
Problem: "I don't want to stop working out."
Solution: Modify, don't halt. Seek guidance from a professional to tailor your workouts to your current capabilities.

The Expert Consultation

3. Seeking Professional Advice:

Strategy:
- Consult with a physiotherapist or fitness professional.
- Gain insights into exercises that promote healing without causing harm.

Troubleshooting Tip:

Problem: "I'm unsure about what exercises are safe."

Solution: A professional assessment provides personalized recommendations for your unique situation.

The Gradual Return

4. Gradual Reintegration of Exercises:

Strategy:

- Slowly reintroduce exercises as your injury heals.
- Gauge your body's response and adjust the intensity accordingly.

Troubleshooting Tip:

Problem: "I want to jump back in at full intensity."

Solution: Patience is key. Gradual reintegration minimizes the risk of re-injury.

The Cross-Training Spectrum

5. Exploring Low-Impact Alternatives:

Strategy:

- Incorporate low-impact activities during the recovery phase.
- Options like swimming, cycling, or yoga can maintain fitness without exacerbating injuries.

Troubleshooting Tip:

Problem: "I miss high-intensity workouts."

Solution: Embrace the opportunity to diversify your training. Low impact doesn't mean low effectiveness.

Your Action Steps:

1. Injury Assessment: Evaluate the severity and nature of your injury.

2. Modification Mastery: Modify workouts to accommodate limitations.

3. Professional Guidance: Consult with a physiotherapist or fitness professional.

4. Slow and Steady Return: Gradually reintroduce exercises with caution.

5. Low-Impact Exploration: Embrace low-impact alternatives during recovery.

Chapter 8

Building a Sustainable Routine

Creating a Long-Term Fitness Plan

Greetings architect of longevity! In this chapter, we're embarking on the crucial mission of building a sustainable fitness routine. It's not just about short-term gains; it's about crafting a routine that stands the test of time, supporting your well-being for the long haul. Let's delve into the art of creating a robust, adaptable, and lifelong fitness plan.

The Blueprint for Longevity

1. Understanding Sustainability:

Insight:
- Sustainability isn't just about immediate results; it's about building habits that endure.
- A sustainable routine should accommodate changes in your life, ensuring fitness remains a constant.

Troubleshooting Tip:
Problem: "I struggle to stick to a routine."
Solution: Reassess your routine. It should be challenging but flexible enough to adapt to life's twists and turns.

The Holistic Approach

2. Incorporating Variety and Balance:

Strategy:
- Include a diverse range of exercises to prevent monotony.
- Balance strength training, cardio, and flexibility work for overall fitness.

Troubleshooting Tip:
Problem: "I get bored easily."
Solution: Variety is the spice of fitness. Try new activities, classes, or outdoor workouts to keep things exciting.

The Realistic Time Investment

3. Tailoring Workouts to Your Schedule:

Strategy:
- Design workouts that fit into your daily life.

- Short, intense sessions can be as effective as longer workouts if consistency is maintained.

Troubleshooting Tip:
Problem: "I don't have time for long workouts."
Solution: Optimize your time. Focus on quality over quantity and find pockets in your day for quick, effective workouts.

The Mind-Body Symbiosis

4. Prioritizing Mental Well-Being:

Strategy:
- Integrate activities that contribute to mental health.
- Yoga, meditation, or outdoor activities can enhance your overall well-being.

Troubleshooting Tip:
Problem: "I'm always stressed."
Solution: Fitness is not just physical. Prioritize activities that bring you joy and peace of mind.

The Adaptive Framework

5. Planning for Life Changes:

Strategy:

- Anticipate life changes and build flexibility into your routine.
- Whether it's travel, work commitments, or family changes, your routine should adapt.

Troubleshooting Tip:

Problem: "Life keeps getting in the way."
Solution: Life is dynamic. Embrace change and modify your routine accordingly, rather than abandoning it.

Your Action Steps:

1. Habitual Integration: Integrate fitness into daily life seamlessly.
2. Routine Refresh: Periodically reassess and refresh your workout routine.
3. Adaptable Framework: Build flexibility to adapt to life changes.
4. Holistic Wellness: Prioritize activities that contribute to mental and emotional well-being.
5. Balanced Variety: Include a mix of exercises for a well-rounded fitness experience.

Balancing Work, Life, and Fitness

Hello life juggler! In this chapter, we're navigating the delicate dance of balancing work, life, and fitness. It's a challenge many face, but fear not; we'll explore practical strategies to harmonize these aspects seamlessly. Let's dive into the art of maintaining equilibrium, ensuring that your fitness journey enhances, rather than hinders, the other vital facets of your life.

The Time Management Tango

1. Strategic Time Allocation:

Insight:
- Balancing work, life, and fitness requires intentional time allocation.
- Identify pockets of time within your day for focused, efficient workouts.

Troubleshooting Tip:
Problem: "I'm too busy for workouts."
Solution: Evaluate your daily schedule. Small, consistent efforts can lead to significant fitness gains.

The Dual-Purpose Duet

2. Integrated Work-Life-Fitness Approach:

Strategy:

- Blend work, life, and fitness when possible.
- Opt for active commuting, walking meetings, or quick workouts during breaks.

Troubleshooting Tip:

Problem: "I struggle to find time for family or social activities."

Solution: Combine activities. Walk with family, do bodyweight exercises with friends, make fitness a social affair.

The Home Workout Harmony

3. Embracing Home Workouts:

Strategy:

- Capitalize on the flexibility of home workouts.
- Choose exercises that don't require extensive equipment and can be done in minimal time.

Troubleshooting Tip:

Problem: "I miss the gym."

Solution: Home workouts can be just as effective. Invest in versatile equipment and recreate the gym vibe at home.

The Motivational Medley

4. Diverse Motivational Tactics:

Strategy:
- Explore various sources of motivation.
- Set personal goals, find a workout buddy, or join virtual fitness communities.

Troubleshooting Tip:
Problem: "I lack motivation."
Solution: Keep it dynamic. Mix up your routine, celebrate small victories, and connect with like-minded individuals for inspiration.

The Consistency Concerto

5. Building Consistent Habits:

Strategy:
- Forge fitness habits that seamlessly integrate into your routine.
- Consistency trumps intensity. Aim for regular, manageable workouts.

Troubleshooting Tip:
Problem: "I struggle to stay consistent."

Solution: Start small, be realistic with your commitments, and gradually increase intensity as habits solidify.

Your Action Steps:

1. Time Treasure Hunt: Identify pockets of time for efficient workouts in your schedule.
2. Integrated Activities: Combine work, life, and fitness activities for synergy.
3. Home Workout Haven: Optimize home workouts for flexibility and convenience.
4. Motivational Mix: Experiment with diverse motivational strategies.
5. Consistency Cornerstone: Build habits that ensure consistent, manageable fitness routines.

Congratulations! You've just mastered the art of balancing work, life, and fitness. In the concluding chapter, we'll explore effective goal-setting strategies and discuss the keys to maintaining a lifelong commitment to your well-being. Get ready to solidify your fitness success!

Conclusion

Congratulations, fitness enthusiast! You've reached the final chapter of "How to Build Muscle Fast With No Equipment: The At-Home Bible For Cutting Gym Costs and Sculpting a Lean Physique Through Calisthenics and Smart Diet Changes." What a journey it's been, from understanding the principles of calisthenics to navigating plateaus, addressing injuries, and seamlessly blending fitness into the tapestry of your life.

As you reflect on the insights, strategies, and actionable steps provided in this guide, remember that your fitness journey is a dynamic, ever-evolving adventure. It's not just about the destination; it's about the continuous pursuit of a stronger, healthier, and more resilient version of yourself.

The Takeaways:

1. Adaptability is Key:
Life changes, and so should your fitness routine. Embrace adaptability as a strength, not a weakness.

2. Consistency Trumps Perfection:
Small, consistent efforts compound into significant results. Every workout, and every healthy meal contributes to your success.

3. Mind and Body Connection:

Fitness isn't just physical; it's a holistic journey. Prioritize mental well-being, and let the benefits resonate throughout your life.

4. Enjoy the Process:

Your fitness journey should be enjoyable. Experiment with workouts, savor nutritious meals and celebrate your victories, big and small.

Your Next Steps:

1. Set Meaningful Goals:

Define clear, achievable goals that align with your aspirations. Your goals are the compass guiding your fitness odyssey.

2. Cultivate a Lifelong Commitment:

Fitness is a lifelong commitment. Approach it with patience, adaptability, and the understanding that it's a journey, not a destination.

3. Stay Connected:

Whether it's with workout buddies, online communities, or fitness professionals, surround yourself with a support system that encourages and motivates.

4. Celebrate Your Progress:
Regularly reflect on how far you've come. Celebrate the milestones, the breakthroughs, and the positive changes in your life.

Your Fitness Odyssey Continues:
This book has equipped you with the tools, strategies, and mindset to sculpt a lean physique, cut gym costs, and embrace the power of calisthenics. As you continue your fitness odyssey, remember that each day is an opportunity to invest in your well-being. Embrace the challenges, savor the victories, and revel in the continuous evolution of your journey.

Thank you for being a part of this fitness adventure. Your commitment to a healthier, stronger you is a journey that echoes far beyond these pages. Here's to your ongoing success, vitality, and the limitless potential within you.

Keep pushing, keep growing, and may your fitness odyssey be an enduring testament to the incredible power you possess.

Wishing you strength, joy, and lifelong well-being,